Asbestos Removal Process, Kit, Bags and Mask

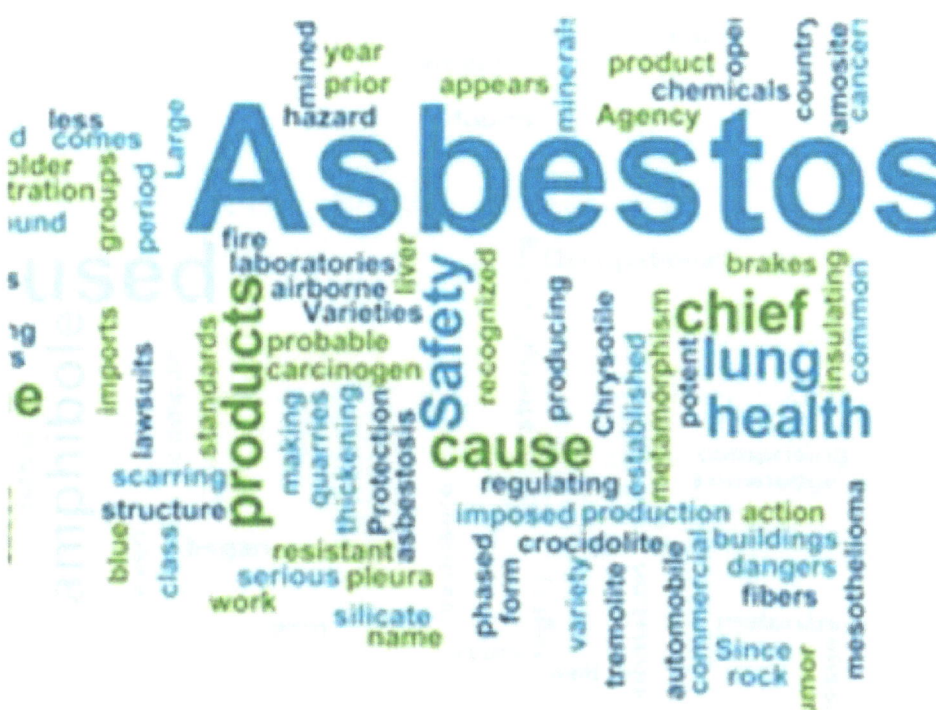

Engr. MD Nursyazwi Bin Mohammad
Greanna Friva Binti Jainal

This e-book was written by

Engr. MD Nursyazwi Bin Mohammad
BEng. (Hons.) Manufacturing Engineering (Design)

And edited by

Greanna Friva Binti Jainal
BA. (Hons.) Education and Science (Chemistry)

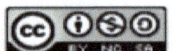
Engr. MD Nursyazwi, Author.
Greanna Friva Jainal, Editor.
P.O.BOX 2073, 90723, Sandakan, Sabah

Vi & Ci Associates

Table of Contents

Meet the Author and the Editor

MEET THE AUTHOR AND EDITOR

The Author

E-book author named Engr. MD Nursyazwi Bin Mohammad, was an entrepreneur in the field of building construction, supplies and services, known generically as Wannah Enterprise. If you are interested, you can visit his website at http://wannah.net/.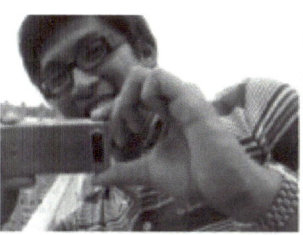

Author comes from Sandakan, Sabah, Malaysia, and is one of the natives in Sabah, Momogun. The writer has a Diploma in Mechanical Engineering (Manufacturing Technology) and Bachelor of Manufacturing Engineering (Manufacturing Design).

Authors have extensive experience in the industry as a Machinist, welder, technician and engineer in some of the leading companies in Malaysia. However, now, active in the business arena.

The Editor

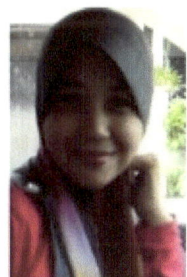 This e-book editor named Greanna Friva Binti Jainal. Editor is a teacher and now serves as an educator at SMK Muhibbah, Sandakan.

Editor is a woman who hails from Sandakan, Sabah, Malaysia. Editor's start higher education in Labuan Matriculation College and then, resume studies in Universiti Malaysia Sabah in the field of Bachelor of Education and Science (Chemistry).

Editor very interested in writing despite busy work in educating students. Editor is also very active in the uniformed units and an Assistant District Commissioner in Sandakan for Scout units.

Chapter 1

Introduction

In this chapter 1, we will get some information about what is asbestos, the effects of Asbestos and where to find Asbestos.

In this ebook we will learn about the asbestos removal process and safeguard yourself against contracting mesothelioma by using a proper Asbestos Removal Kit, Asbestos Removal Bags and also Asbestos Removal Mask.

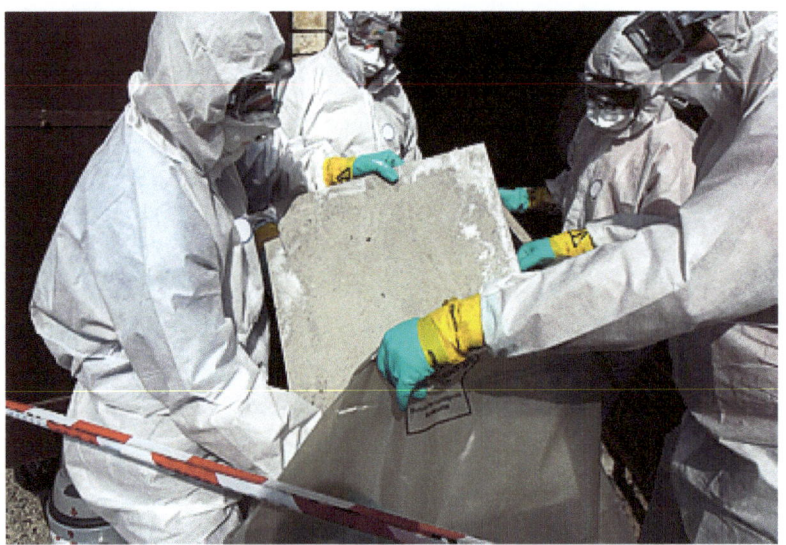

For further step, we will go through this ebook together.

What is Asbestos?

Asbestos as we know, often linked to mesothelioma, a rare form of cancer but can be fatal, ie by, stimulates tumor growth of a layer that surrounds the vital organs.

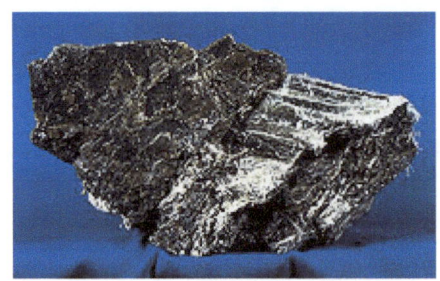

Asbestos from WikiPedia "saying",

Asbestos is a set of six naturally occurring silicate minerals used commercially for their desirable physical properties.

They all have in common their eponymous, asbestiform habit: long (ca. 1:20 aspect ratio), thin fibrous crystals. The prolonged inhalation of asbestos fibers can cause serious illnesses including malignant lung cancer, mesothelioma, and asbestosis (a type of pneumoconiosis). The European Union has banned all use of asbestos, as well as the extraction, manufacture, and processing of asbestos products.

Asbestos mining began more than 4,000 years ago, but did not start large-scale until the end of the 19th century. For a long time, the world's largest asbestos mine was the Jeffrey mine in the town of Asbestos, Quebec.

Asbestos was not used in construction today, but, still known embodied in many ancient structures, including schools and factories which have long operated.

Effects of Asbestos

Although not harmful to causing emotional distress, however, we are still shackled because we still find that many buildings still contain hazardous materials, the fibers can be dispersed in the air, either during project construction or accidents (such as fire or earthquake).

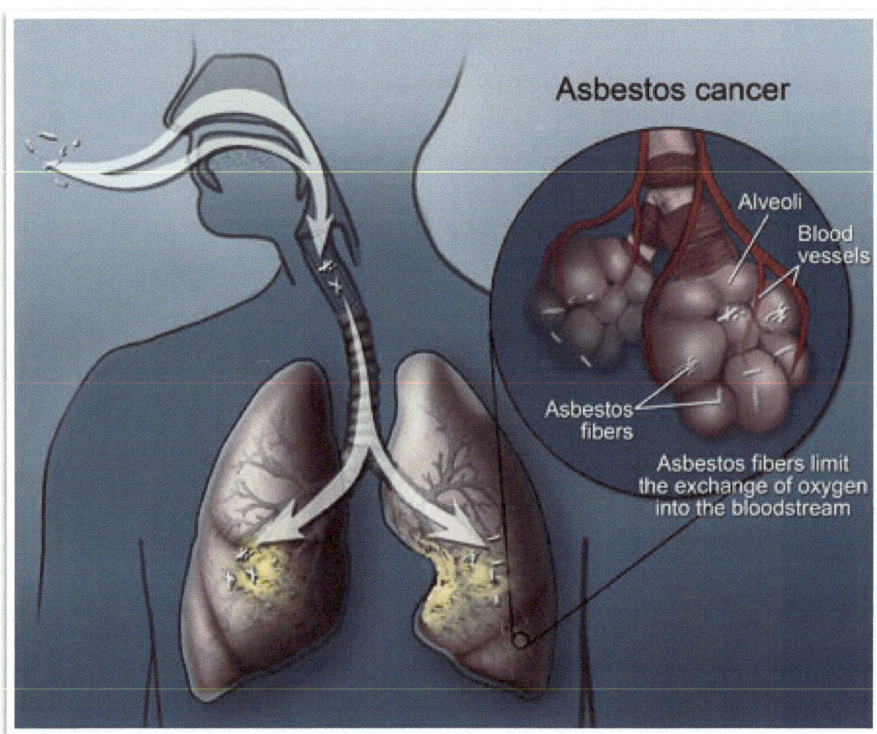

If you know your home or your business store structure contains asbestos, it may take some time to remove it. Asbestos removal process is very long and complex.

Special measures should be taken immediately to eliminate the possibility of the release of asbestos fibers into the air. If such cases occur, the asbestos fibers will place all life at risk for mesothelioma.

Where to find Asbestos?

The fibers are difficult to detect because they are microscopic and can not be felt in any case a particular scent or taste. Risks involved in the process of removing asbestos recently been the subject of a very tense debate.

But lets see the picture below.

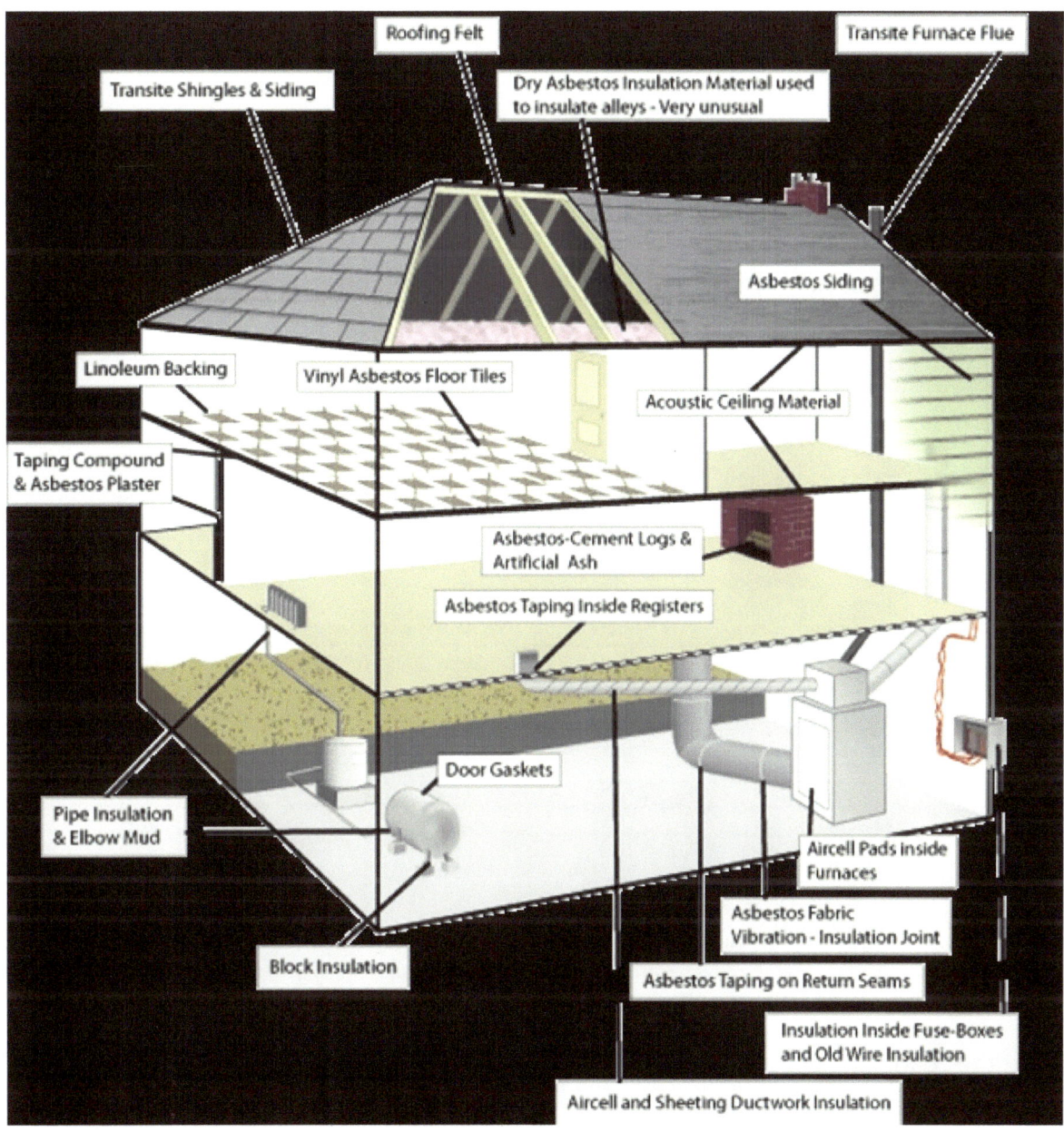

This is some possiblities you might located where Asbestos is.

Chapter 2

Safe Asbestos Removal Process

Before we start the Asbestos Removal Process, the best way is to buy any approved asbestos plastic bag and send the sample to test.

Asbestos Removal Test Kit

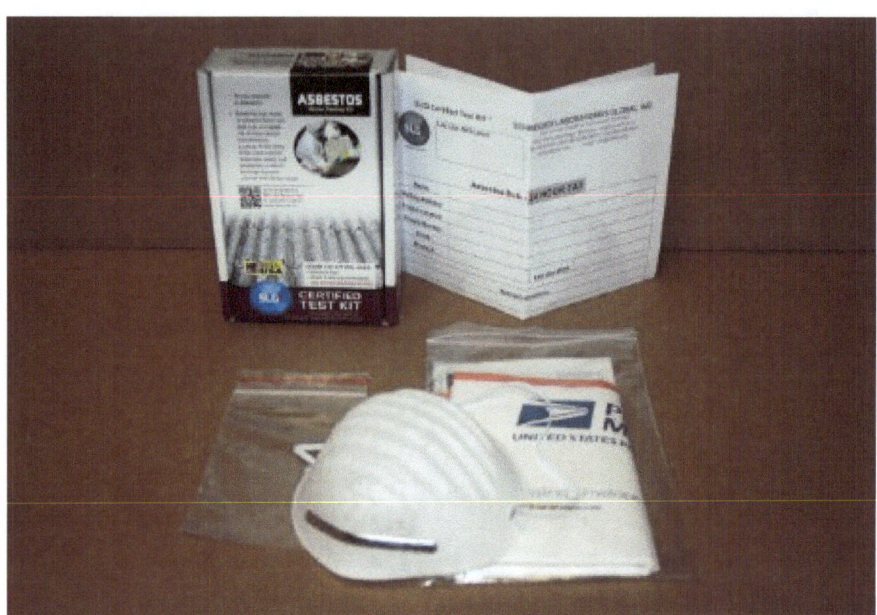

Click here for Asbestos Removal Test Kit

If the results positive, you should continue the next step.

The following steps ensure that asbestos-containing material is removed safely, that the removal process provides a clean environment, and that asbestos removal jobs meet or exceed California's Department of Toxic Substance Control (DTSC) requirements for asbestos removal.

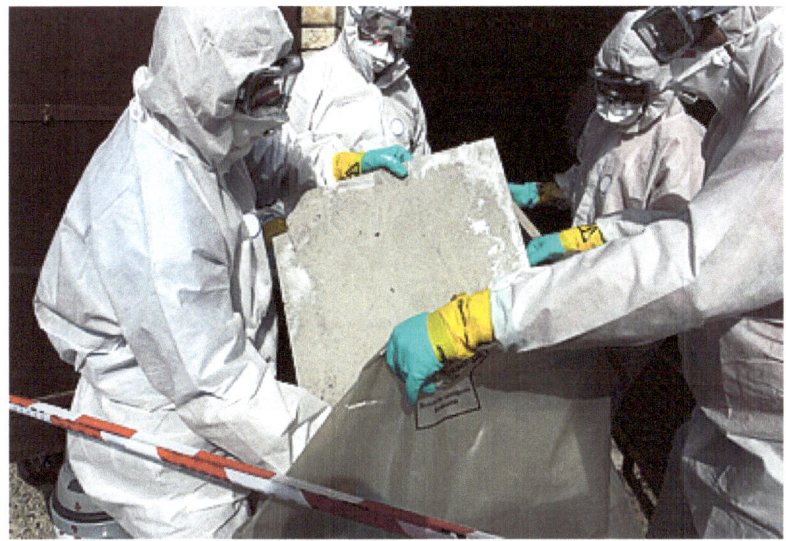

Each step ensures the health and safety of our workers and others who will enter the removal area after abatement.

Step 1: Setting Up an Asbestos Containment

Safe asbestos removal process should start with, cover the areas where we want to do the work, which is a place with asbestos containing materials.

You should cover the contaminated surface with 6 mil plastic sheeting. Plastic sheets keep dust and asbestos fibers from entering into another area or room structure.

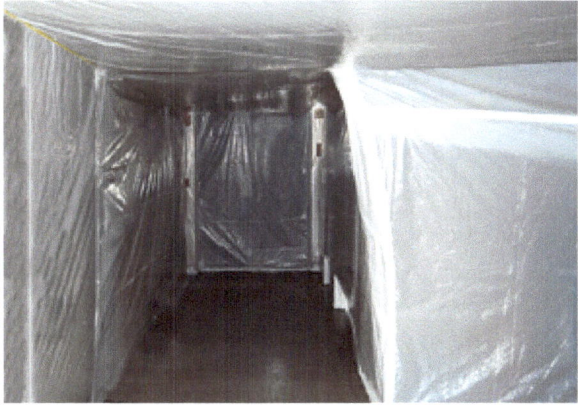

Control zone should be configured to meet the specific needs during the removal of asbestos. You should pay special attention to windows, doors, countertop, cabinets, sink, shower and tub to ensure that no asbestos dust can contact any of the accessories.

After the formation of a buffer zone, check the seal attached to ensure that asbestos fibers can not escape from the containment area.

Then put HEPA machine turned negative three stages in the work area and installation of air duct cleaning production. Negative HEPA filter machines that have been stored in the exhaust pipe and fresh air out, while trapping airborne particles of asbestos vacuum filter.

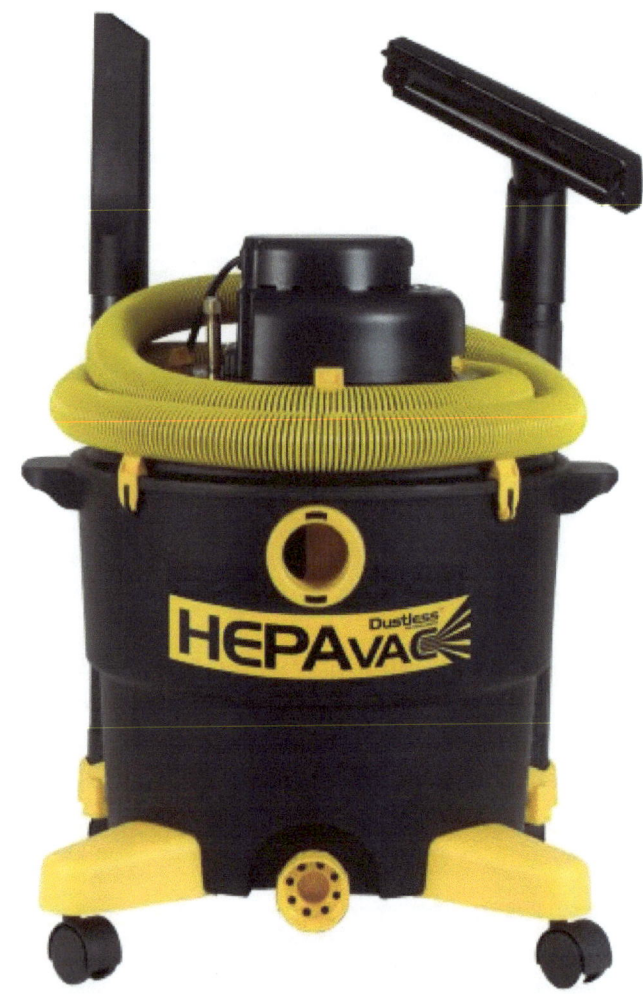

Click here for 16-Gallon Dustless Wet/Dry Vacuum with Hepa Filter

Finally, we ensure that all asbestos removal equipment and tools with a bit of work in place ready to be used in place of control.

Step 2: Wearing equipment such as a Respirator and Protective Suit

Before we begin asbestos removal work, we MUST wear protective clothing made of material called Tyvek. You also MUST wear a special respirator for asbestos removal and material should be of high quality.

Asbestos Removal Protective Wear made from Tyvek

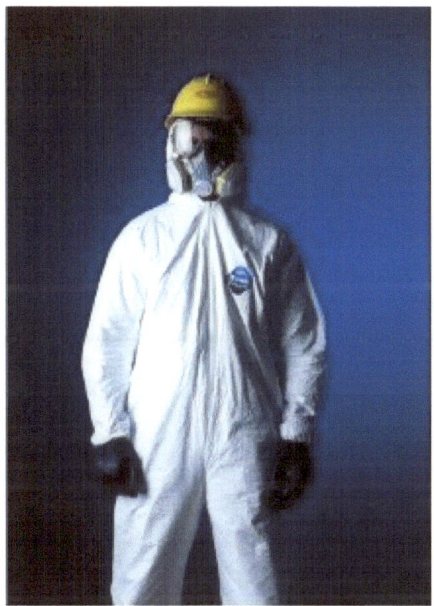

Click here to know more about this Protective Clothing

Asbestos Removal Protective Clothing

- Serged seams, attached hood, front zipper closure, elastic wrists, and attached boots.
- Inherent barrier protection against dry particulate hazards.
- Applications range from agriculture to spray painting to lead remediation.
- Even after abrasions, stops microporous particles better than other reusable garments.
- The best balance of protection, durability and comfort.

Asbestos Removal Mask or Respirator

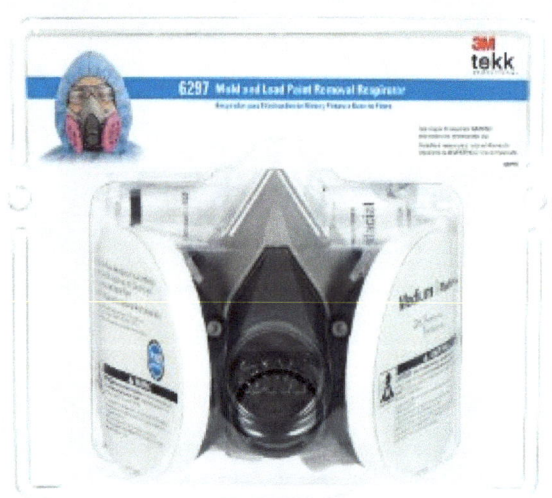

Click here to know more about this Respirator

Asbestos Removal Mask

- Use for mold remediation in accordance with US-EPA Guidelines and sanding and scraping lead-based paint
- For workplace/occupational applications only
- Helps reduce exposure to mold spores and odors
- Important educational information included
- NIOSH approved: P100

Step 3: Closed Entry to Work Area and Start Negative Air Machine

Close and secure the entry to the work area prior to starting to remove asbestos-containing material. After the asbestos removal process begins, no unauthorized person shall be allowed enter the work area.

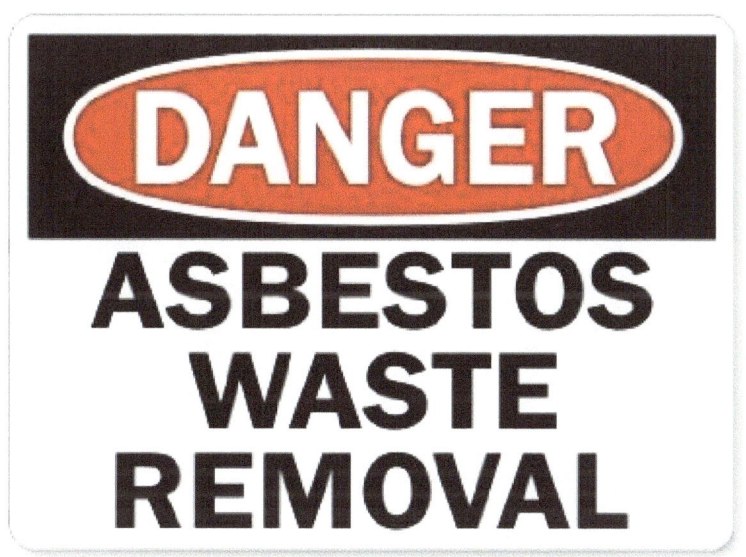

Click here for Asbestos Removal Warning Sign

Before removing any asbestos-containing material, turn on the three-stage HEPA negative air machine. Make sure the air ducts installed on the machine are running to the outside.

Step 4: Asbestos Removal Bags As Asbestos Removal Proceeds

Depending on the type of material being removed, place the removed material in containers.

As you remove asbestos containing material, you should spray the material with water amended with an approved surfactant.

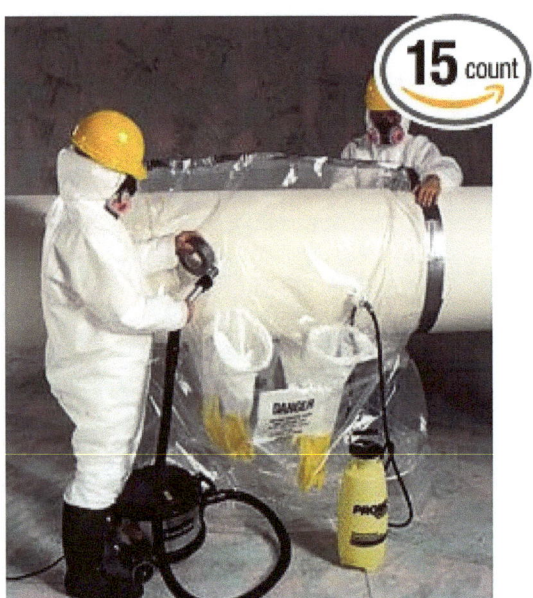

When the material is wet on all sides, we put the material in double bags 6 mil thick. Then we seal each bag assembly conforming with requirements before we start filling another bag.

Step 5: Clean Area After Asbestos Removed

After finished succesfully removing the asbestos-containing material, you MUST clean the abated area with HEPA vacuum cleaners and clean wet rags.

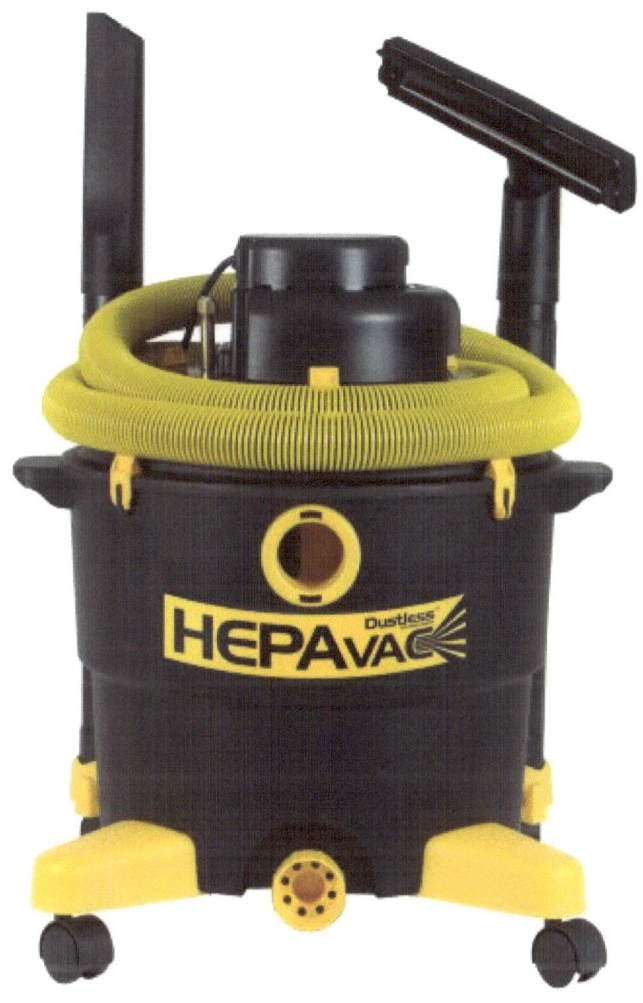

Click here for 16-Gallon Dustless Wet/Dry Vacuum with Hepa Filter

At the same time, you should dispose of the cleaning rags in double 6-mill bags in the same manner that we disposed of the asbestos-containing material.

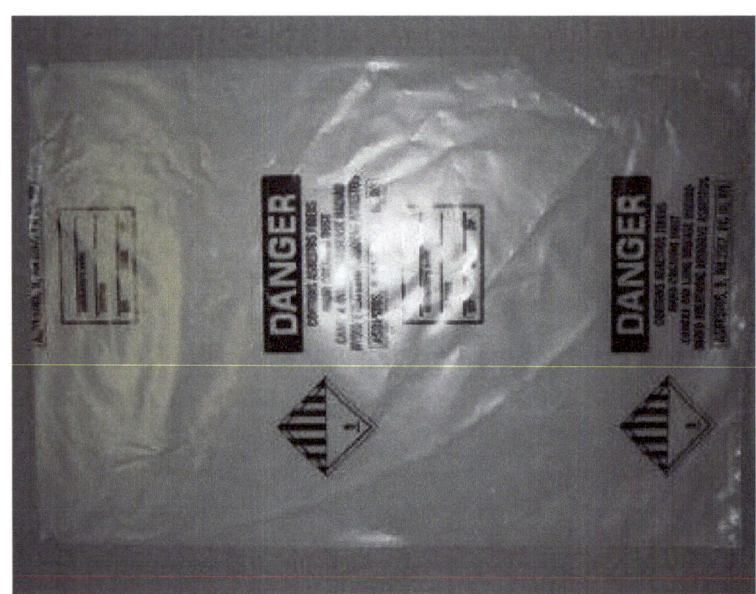

Click here for 6 Mil Poly Disposable Bags Printed With Asbestos Warning

Step 6: Dispose Your Protective Clothing

At the end of the job, you should remove the protective tyvek suit and dispose of the tyvek suit in a double plastic bag and seal the bag.

Below is a disposable protective suit. Therefore you don't need to put it inside double plastic bag to reduce cost. But, you still can do it for safety precaution.

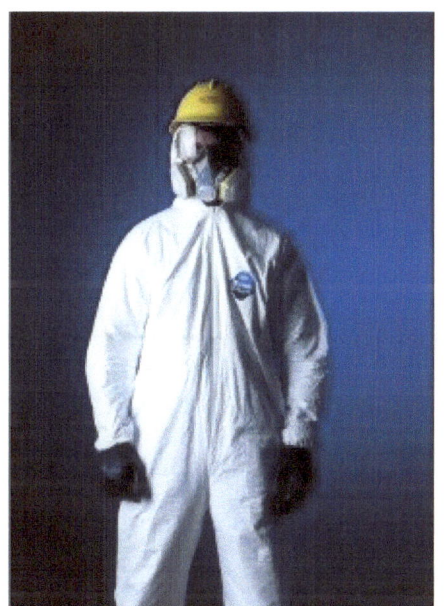

Click here to know more about this Protective Clothing

Chapter 3

Conclusions

Many companies all over the world get the initiative to remove asbestos from buildings that are dilapidated.

Whereas, the government even be involved in contracts with companies to remove asbestos. The controversy around the removal is not likely disappear any time soon.

However, people will start to understand that the higher risk may arise if there are still individuals who want to maintain asbestos as is.

Finally, it is their choice to prepare specific equipment if there are individuals who want to remove the asbestos found in the structure. Although this decision is not always easy, but it is very necessary to do.

I hope you can benefited from this ebook about Asbestos Removal Process and the equipment involved as given before such as Asbestos Removal Bags, Asbestos Removal Respirator, Asbestos Removal Kit, Asbestos Removal Protective Clothing and many more.

Thank You

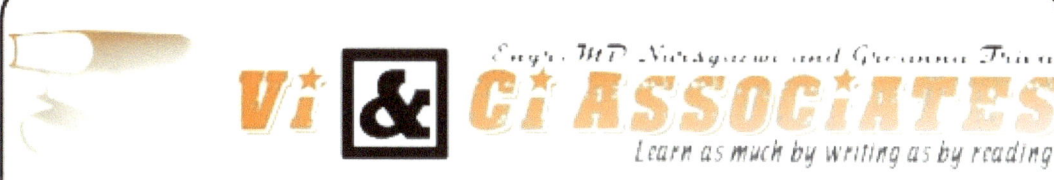

This e-book was written by

Engr. MD Nursyazwi Bin Mohammad
BEng. (Hons.) Manufacturing Engineering (Design)

And edited by

Greanna Friva Binti Jainal
BA. (Hons.) Education and Science (Chemistry)

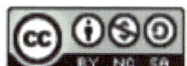

Visit Us

For more information about **Vi & Ci Associates**, you can visit us at
http://wannah.net/blog/vi-ci-associates

OR

Scan this QR Code